Plagiocephaly & Torticollis:
Tips from a Pediatric Physical Therapist

Whitney Castle, PT, DPT

I would like to thank my husband and daughter for allowing me to take extra time to write this book, even though most of my time spent writing this was after our daughter was asleep! They are both very supportive of my ideas on how to help other babies and children through my PT career. Thank you also to God for giving me the confidence and knowledge to complete this book.

Table of Contents

About the Author

Whitney is a graduate of the East Tennessee State University Doctorate of Physical Therapy Program. Since graduating and passing her state licensing board, she has worked in several physical therapy settings. The majority of her work has been with the pediatric population working with developmental delays, the special needs population, plagiocephaly, torticollis and early intervention.

She is a wife, mother to a 4-year-old little princess, and 9-year-old dog, Duke. In her free time, she enjoys attending church, spending time with family, doing "stretches" aka yoga with her daughter, going to the beach and Disney, and watching movies as a family.

Her goal is to help educate parents, families, daycare staff, and other health professionals on the importance of early intervention for the baby and child in any aspect of their growing life including plagiocephaly, torticollis, and gross motor milestones.

Chapter 1
What is Positional Plagiocephaly and How to Detect It?

Positional plagiocephaly, also known as flat head syndrome, is when a baby develops a flattening on the back or side of the head. If left untreated, babies with plagiocephaly may develop vision problems and asymmetries of the head and face. (1) This can be caused by the baby's position inside the womb or can occur after the baby is born for other reasons. After birth, the baby can acquire torticollis due congenital muscle tightness (rare), positioning in the womb, or preferring to look to one side. Any of these reasons can affect the shape of the baby's head since their skull is malleable, which allows the skull (and fontanels/sutures) to shift and expand for the rapidly growing brain. Sometimes there are also facial asymmetries that occur with plagiocephaly which can affect the forehead, cheeks, and ears. Picture the skull as a balloon. When squeezed, it affects the other areas that are not being pushed. This is the same as the skull. If one spot is flat (like the back of the head), the opposite side (such as the forehead) may be "pushed out." There are several types of flat head syndrome that usually depend on how the baby is positioned or prefers to turn his/her head. There are also different severity levels of the flatness for each type. Here are some examples.

Plagiocephaly means "oblique head". Some characteristics are:
- Head is flat on one side
- One ear is more forward than the other
- One eye is smaller than the other
- One cheek is fuller than the other
- Top of the head is not level
- One side of the forehead is more forward

Below is a representation of plagiocephaly on the right side of the skull, although there may be different cases, such as mild or more severe cases.

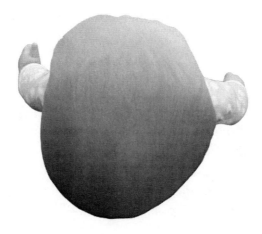

Brachycephaly means "short head". The back of the head becomes flat, causing an abnormally wide, tall head shape. Some characteristics are:
- Head is wider than normal
- Head is abnormally tall
- Back of head is flat rather than curved
- The face appears small relative to the size of the head
- The widest part of the head is just above the ears (2)

Below is a representation of brachycephaly shaped head, although there may be different cases, such as mild or more severe cases.

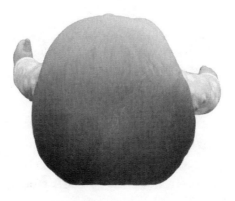

For comparison, here is a representation of a normal shaped head.

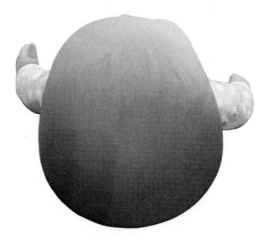

Taking pictures of the baby's head with hair wet is an easy way to detect any flat spots. The pictures can also be used to compare the baby's head shape each week or month.

Chapter 2
Preventing Plagiocephaly

Prevention is key when it comes to keeping your baby's head shape from getting flat. The peak prevalence of developmental plagiocephaly is 4 months of age because an infant is not able to hold his or her head up when sitting without support and has little active positioning of the head; at 6 months, the infant should have strong and steady head control. In his or her first 6 months, an infant's head grows rapidly. (3)

Positioning, or how the baby is held or placed on a flat surface, is very important in preventing the risk of plagiocephaly. The baby should be given ample floor when not sleeping, which gives the baby the opportunity to freely move around. When sleeping, the baby should be placed in the supine position (on their back) until the age of 1 year old. The American Academy of Pediatrics recommends that parents place the baby on his or her back during sleep which reduces the risk of SIDS (Sudden Infant Death Syndrome.)(4)

Now, once the baby learns how to roll over this may be easier said than done. You may be waking up more to check to see if he or she is on their tummy, which adds to those sleepless nights. Roll the baby to his or her back or if they are old enough to roll from back to belly and belly to back, let them decide which position they want to sleep. Babies that can roll over (usually around 4-6 months) are at a decreased risk of SIDS. Alternating the baby's head to the right and left during sleep can help decrease the risk of developing a flat spot. When the supine position is necessary, such as during sleeping, unhindered movement should be encouraged. This includes avoiding prolonged time in a car seat, baby swing, and other carriers. In addition, alter the position of items of interest frequently, such as by rotating toys from side to side or by alternating the direction the baby is facing. (5) During awake time, the baby should be given plenty of supervised tummy time (time on his or her stomach) to allow the back of his or her head relief from the pressure of lying down on a flat surface. This position also helps strengthen his or her neck and shoulder muscles.

There are several ways to incorporate tummy time activities, even if the baby does not prefer this position. These activities will be discussed in another chapter. It is important to remember that since the baby's head is very malleable, that the baby should not be placed in one position for any extended period of time. Sometimes placing the baby in swings or bouncy seats can be helpful during household tasks or caring for other children. However, the longer the baby is kept in the same position, the risk of developing flat spots and torticollis increases over time.

Floortime is the best opportunity for the baby to explore and learn how their whole body will move in their environment. The baby has more opportunity to move their head, arms, hands, trunk, legs, and feet while lying on the floor. As always, floor time should be supervised at any age to avoid the risk of injury with their surroundings. Baby gates that can be connected to make a shape, pack and plays, or playpens can also be very useful to allow the baby to move more freely.

Babywearing is another option that can help prevent and improve flat head the baby is having difficulty adjusting to positioning during awake time. Babywearing allows the baby's head to move freely and look around at surroundings. It also removes the pressure of a surface pushing on the back of the side of the head.

Chapter 3
Tummy Time and Activities

Research found that if infants were placed to sleep on their stomachs, their risk of dying from SIDS increased by at least two-fold.

As a result, the "Back-to-Sleep" Campaign was initiated in 1994 with a focus to encourage parents to put their babies to sleep on their backs to reduce the risk of SIDS. After starting the "Back-to-Sleep" campaign, the number of deaths due to SIDS have dramatically decreased. (6)

Since the start of the "Back-to-Sleep" campaign, the importance of increased tummy time has also gained popularity with parents and healthcare professionals to offset the amount of time and pressure that is put on the baby's head.

Here are some activities to help make tummy time more fun for everyone. Some may work instantly, and some will work overtime. There is no specific order in which these steps should be used. However, all of these steps have one thing in common... they work! You have to take the first step to help your baby's head shape and movement. Take 5 minutes to read this guide to help improve your baby's head shape and movement.

Without knowing your baby's type, severity, or history of plagiocephaly and/or torticollis, I cannot tell you which of these will work best for you. Also, there are no guarantees that any one thing will work. But over the last 7 years, I've been able to narrow down what does and does not work when it comes to decreasing plagiocephaly and torticollis.

These 7 steps are included among the steps that do work. But imagine this...how great it would be if you could just try one of these tips every day.

Within a few weeks, you could have all 7 of these easy steps working for you and your baby – giving you more time to play and enjoy your baby's milestones.
⏰
Take time to add at least one of these steps to your daily routine. It won't take long and they will only cost you a few minutes of your day. I think you will be amazingly surprised at how easy they are to incorporate into your daily routine.

1) Playtime on tummy.

There are several ways to incorporate tummy time into the daily routine and make it fun for both you and the baby. Tummy time should always be supervised and during awake time. Tummy time includes any position that allows the back of the baby's head to be relieved of any pressure. The position also allows the neck and back muscles to strengthen. Tummy time does not always have to be completely flat on the floor. It can include using boppy pillows, regular pillows, or rolled-up towels if the baby does not like being completely flat during tummy time initially. You can keep the baby happy and entertained by using mirrors, toys, books and even getting down on the floor with the baby so he or she can see your face. Also, you can try lying the baby on different textures of blankets. Here are a few pictures of tummy time.

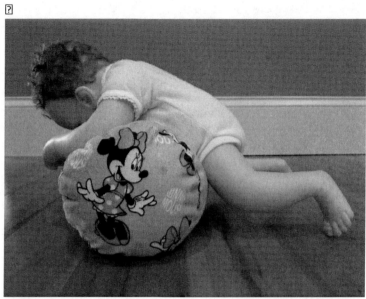

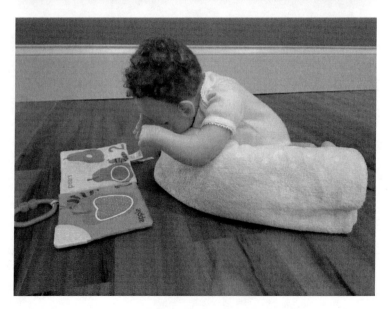

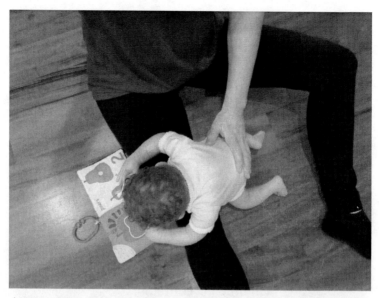

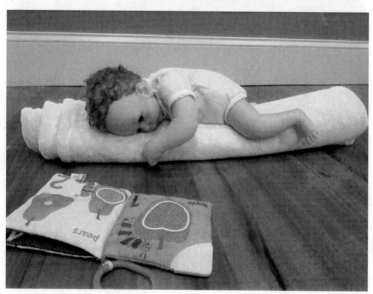

2) Roll baby onto tummy after diaper changes.

One of the easiest ways to incorporate tummy time into your daily routine is to include it after a diaper change. We all know how many diapers babies go through during the day! This is especially helpful if the baby is not a fan of tummy time. After you change the diaper, roll the baby over on his or her tummy for 30 seconds to 1 minute. This is a good starting point to try to make it more enjoyable for you and the baby. You can later work up to 1-5 minutes. Now, this does not have to be after every diaper change, but it is an easy step to add. ⏺

3. Avoid too much time in "containers."

This step is not a position for tummy time, but it is a very important step for the baby's muscles and development. "Containers" are items like car seats, swings, exersaucers, and rockers. These items are fine to place the baby in while trying to get yourself ready, cook dinner, shower, clean, or help them to fall asleep. However, too much time in these types of equipment does not allow the baby to freely move his or her head, neck, or body during sleep or awake time. Babies should not be left to sleep in these to prevent injury.

4. Tummy time on you!

This is probably my favorite step! You and the baby will probably agree, especially during those first few weeks and months where the baby likes being held. Again, tummy time does not have to be flat on the floor. Carrying your baby in your arms with their head at your shoulder is a great way to help strengthen the neck muscles and allows the back of the head to not be against a surface. You can also lie on the floor or bed with the baby on your chest. This allows the baby to see your face and try to raise his or her head off your chest to strengthen the neck muscles. ⏹

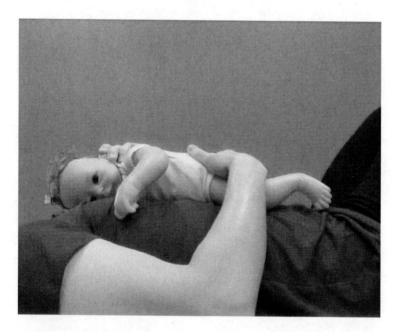

5. Side-Lying position.

The side-lying position is a great alternative to tummy time, especially if the baby is not a fan of tummy time or has plagiocephaly (flat head syndrome). This position will help the baby get used to different positions other than lying on his or her back. Side-lying also allows the back of the head to not be compressed on a surface, which will help in shaping his or her head if it is flat on one side. This position also helps with rolling over if the baby is ready for that skill. The picture below is for reference of side-lying position, and the baby should be supervised in side-lying position in awake or sleep time.

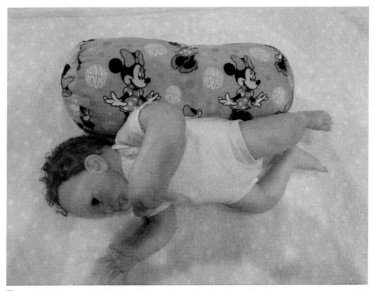

?

6. Football carry

The football carry or airplane carry is a fun way to incorporate tummy time. This carry is very helpful if the baby starts to get fussy or likes to be carried. While holding the baby in your arms, you will place the baby on his or her tummy on your forearms/arms using one of both of your arms. In this position, you can stand in front of a mirror and allow the baby to look at him/herself. You can also bounce or swing the baby in this position and make it even more fun or relaxing. This picture is used for reference of football carry, and the baby should be awake and supervised during tummy time activities.

14

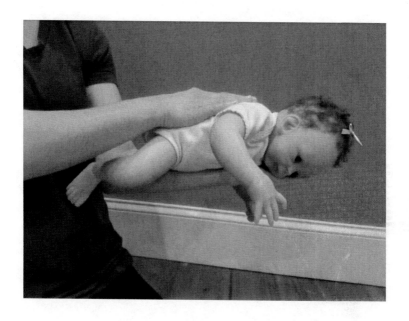

7. See a Physical Therapist in your area!

There isn't any quicker way to improve the baby's plagiocephaly and/or torticollis than to see a good physical therapist. Going to see a hands-on specialized physical therapist means you're going to get fast access to someone who knows how to help you and the baby improve his/her head shape and movement. Physical therapists, especially those specialized in pediatrics, know how to help you and the baby find ways to incorporate tummy time and positioning into your daily routine.

Usually, you will leave your physical therapist after the first session feeling less concerned and stressed!

Follow all the steps combined with a trip to see a good, hands-on physical therapist and you will see a dramatic drop in the plagiocephaly and/or torticollis you are currently experiencing with your baby

Chapter 4
Early Intervention is Key

Early intervention is key when it comes to preventing and treating plagiocephaly and torticollis, which sometimes occurs along with plagiocephaly.

In my experience as a pediatric physical therapist, there are more treatable cases when the baby was referred and treated as soon as plagiocephaly or torticollis has been detected, by parent or pediatrician. It is much easier to implement and adjust positioning and tummy time activities at 2 or 3 months of age instead of 5 or 6 months of age. Once the infant starts moving more and possibly rolling, usually past 3 months of age, positioning activities can be more challenging. The purpose of positioning activities is to avoid pressure on the back or side of the head for prolonged periods. Therefore, if the baby starts moving more and not staying in the position they were placed in, then the progress can take longer or may require other options. Helmets are another option and will be discussed in a later chapter.

Through my career, I have heard parents and pediatricians say to "wait and see" or "he/she will grow out of it." These statements may very well be true, however, the cases that I have treated usually do not have the same progress when referred later. The longer the wait between detection and treatment, the longer it may take for the flattening to improve.

If you believe the baby needs treatment for plagiocephaly and/or torticollis and the pediatrician says to "wait and see," please request a physical therapy referral for evaluation or change pediatricians. There is nothing wrong with getting a second opinion when it comes to your baby. Even though it may seem more of a cosmetic issue, long term effects of plagiocephaly and torticollis can affect vision as well as wearing eyeglasses, hats, and sports helmets. Eyeglasses, hats, and sports helmets may not fit or feel like they fit right when there is still flattening on the head. Also, if the child wants or has to wear short hair, it may not look the same as others. The child will thank you later for improving their head shape.

Chapter 5
Torticollis

The term torticollis is derived from the Latin words Tortus for twisted and collum for the neck. Torticollis is classified as either congenital (present at birth) or acquired (occurring later in infancy or childhood). The most common type is congenital muscular torticollis. Sometimes it is hard to notice until children are several weeks old, once they start to gain more control of their head movement. (7)

Congenital muscular torticollis can be treated with physical therapy, especially when it's started early. There's that "early intervention is key" I've been talking about! it is associated with plagiocephaly.

Acquired torticollis typically occurs in the first 4 to 6 months of childhood or later. Typically, there is usually no facial asymmetry with acquired torticollis. Acquired torticollis can be benign (not serious) or a sign of more serious health issues. Because the causes can be so different, it is very important to act quickly so that your child can get the proper care and treatment. Therefore, I will discuss congenital torticollis through the remainder of this book.

An infant with torticollis will tilt their head to one side, and sometimes the chin will tilt upwards. It looks like the infant is tilting their ear to their shoulder, and the chin points upwards. This can happen because of positioning in the womb or preferring to look to one side after birth, which is why it can be associated with plagiocephaly.

The best way to determine if your infant has torticollis is to get an assessment by the pediatrician and/or physical therapist, preferably one who specializes in pediatrics. Again, if you feel that your infant or toddler has torticollis and the pediatrician says "to wait and see", ask for a physical therapy referral or request a second opinion.

Here are some activities to include in helping to correct torticollis. These are not to disregard exercises or interventions given by another physical therapist but may be used in conjunction or used if in the "wait and see" boat.

In order to help relieve the tension in the tight neck muscle, you will be moving the infant's head to each side and more so to the tight side.

Example: An infant has a hard time looking to the right, turn the infant's head to that side with little overpressure, not too hard.

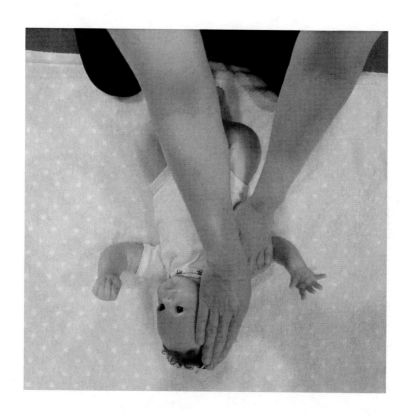

Side-lying during playtime is an excellent way to incorporate stretching the affected muscle and helps to strengthen the affected muscle because the infant might try to lift their head off the support surface. This position also helps with bringing hands together, hands to mouth, and playing with toys.

Prone, or tummy time, with head turned to the affected side (right side tight, right ear is on support surface/floor/blanket) will help to stretch the tight muscle and also help strengthen neck and shoulder muscles. Tummy time for the win again! Another option that also goes with plagiocephaly is changing the side the infant is fed from, whether breastfeeding or bottle-feeding. Both sides are used during breastfeeding, but the infant might feed better or prefer one side more than the other.

Aside from preferring to look to one side, an infant with torticollis might also prefer other activities or movements to one side or avoid one side altogether. This is when it is important to help your baby to use both sides in all movements that babies go through like using both hands, both legs, and rolling. A good way to incorporate this into your daily routine is to move both their hands overhead like "stretching to the sky" or "So Big." Another activity is helping your baby reach and grab for the toes with their hands by moving their feet towards their hands. You can sing songs during this movement like "Row, row, row your boat" to make it more fun!

Trunk rotation, or turning their belly/back to either side is very helpful when learning to roll and can be difficult if your baby has torticollis due to the muscles in the neck and upper back being tight. You can help your baby with trunk rotation by turning their upper body towards one side while they are in a supported sitting position like the picture below (with very little overpressure as to not force the movement).

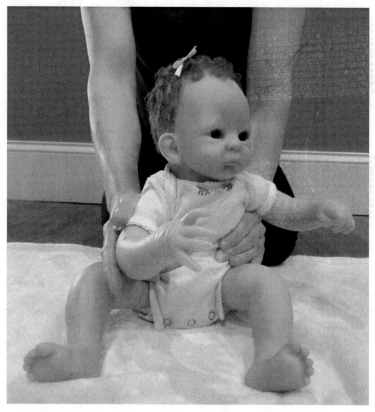

It is very important to remember placement of toys while playing so that infant is giving opportunity to look to the opposite side of the affected tight muscle. This is also true during feeding, such as placing yourself to the affected side so that baby attempts to look at towards the food. Infants are all about symmetry (same on each side) after 2-3 months of age. The infant needs to be able to roll to both sides, look to both directions, use both arms and legs equally, and grab both feet with each hand. This helps for later development with crawling, walking, going up/downstairs, running, jumping jacks and bicycling...any movement where both sides are being used at the same time.

Chapter 6
Helmet Options and Tips

A helmet or cranial helmet is another option to help treat plagiocephaly. As a pediatric physical therapist, I always mention this during an evaluation of the baby for plagiocephaly, whether the baby will need it or not. I like to inform the parents or caregivers of all the options, especially with thoughts that usually come with a helmet. Most parents say they want to avoid getting a helmet or they do not want to have their baby wear a helmet because of negative comments. However, the thought process needs to be shifted towards the baby's future if the helmet would have helped but was avoided and now the child has difficulty wearing glasses, baseball caps, sports helmets, or different hairstyles. Most of the time, if the plagiocephaly is caught early, usually around 2-4 months, then positioning activities work to improve and correct the flattening. However, if the plagiocephaly is treated after 4-6 months of age, it is more difficult to correct the flattening and other methods of treatment are needed, like a helmet.

The baby usually wears the helmet approximately 23 hours a day for a few months, depending on the severity and when the baby was referred for therapy or helmet assessment. Collett, et al (2011), found that toddlers with plagiocephaly continue to exhibit developmental delays compared to toddlers without plagiocephaly, especially in the areas of cognition and language. (9)

There are a few cranial helmet companies, like Cranial Technologies including DOC Band, and STARBand. The baby will most likely need a physician referral for an assessment by an orthotist that offers cranial helmets. The orthotist will provide an assessment of the baby's head shape usually with a computer scanner to get a 3-D image. The cranial helmet is made, fitted to baby, and adjustments can be made if needed during the treatment process depending on the progress of the head shape.

Several support groups can be found to help with wearing, cleaning, and decorating helmets, as well as additional tips from personal experience provided by other parents or caregivers.

Chapter 7
Additional Activities

Also, you can follow me on Facebook and Instagram under PedsPTMentor. Thank you.

Football carry previously mentioned.

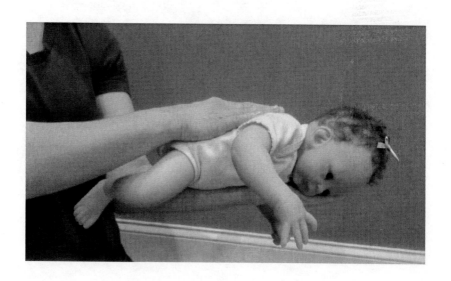

Side-lying with support from rolled-up towel or pillow.

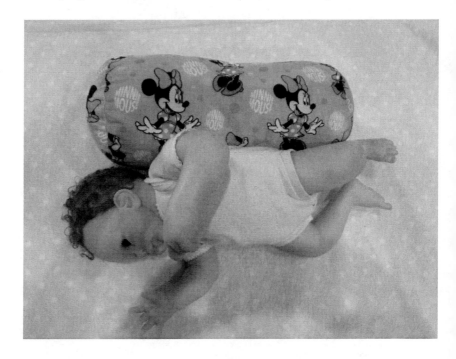

Tummy Time options.

Tummy time over rolled-up towel or bolster pillow.

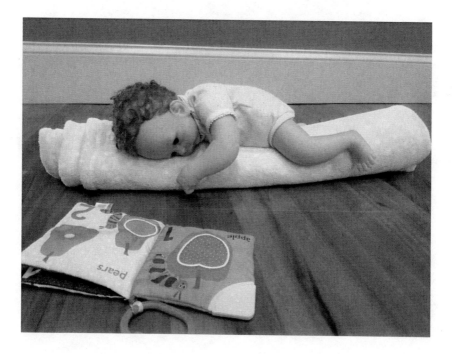

Tummy time over boppy pillow, rolled-up towel, or soft bolster.

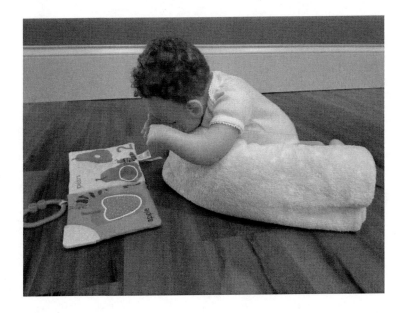

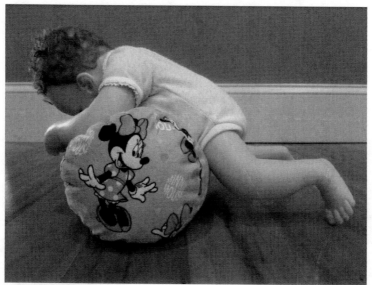

Washcloth/towel roll around head to be used during awake hours or supervised sleep (similar to Tortle cap). This help prevents baby turning to affected side, keep head in midline or giving opportunity to look in non-affected side.

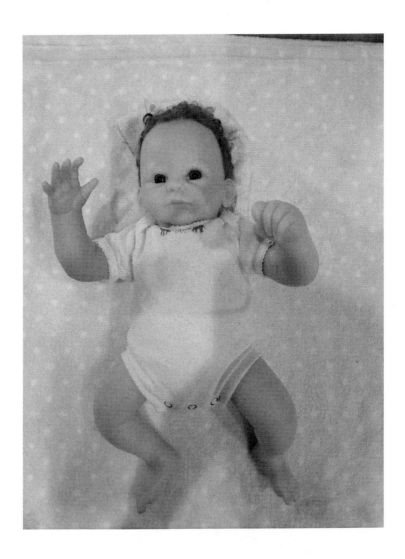

References

1) https://pathways.org/positional-plagiocephaly-positional-torticollis/
2) https://www.cranialtech.com/plagiocephaly/
3) Evidence-Based Care of the Child With Deformational Plagiocephaly, Part I: Assessment and Diagnosis.

Looman, Wendy S. et al. Journal of Pediatric Health Care, Volume 26, Issue 4, 242 - 250

4) SIDS and Other Sleep-Related Infant Deaths: Updated 2016 Recommendations for a Safe Infant Sleeping Environment. TASK FORCE ON SUDDEN INFANT DEATH SYNDROME. Pediatrics Nov 2016, 138 (5) e20162938; DOI: 10.1542/peds.2016-2938

5) Deformational Plagiocephaly: A guide to Diagnosis and Treatment. Boston Children's Hospital: Plastic and Oral Surgery. Interactive PDF #3084. 1-16.

6) https://www.aap.org/en-us/advocacy-and-policy/aap-health-initiatives/7-great-achievements/Pages/Reducing-Sudden-Infant-Death-with-Back-to-.aspx

7) http://www.childrenshospital.org/conditions-and-treatments/conditions/t/torticollis

8) Collet B, Starr J, Kartin D, Heike C, Berg J, Cunningham M, Speltz M. Development in Toddlers with and without deformational plagiocephaly. Arch Pediatr Adolesc Med. 2011 Jul; 165(7):653-658.

Made in United States
Cleveland, OH
13 July 2025

18533369R00024